MAN

Vs

PROSTRATE:

100% Ageing Secret

Dr. Ben Chapman

Dr. Ben Chapman

Man Vs Prostrate

Dr. Ben Chapman

INTRODUCTION
CHAPTER ONE

CHAPTER THREE

The Relationship between Physical Activity and BPH

How Much Exercise Should I Do if I'm Concerned about my Prostate Health?

What Is My Heart Rate?

Smart Fitness Club

Bicycle Saddle and Health

Choose a spacious area with plenty of padding.

Aerobic Exercise - Pick Your Favorite Activities

Exercise   safely

Man Vs Prostrate

INTRODUCTION

Personal care guide. Patients face a real dilemma when choosing between several treatments with potentially irreversible consequences. Research shows that partially informed treatment choices often lead to regret.

When you are first diagnosed with prostate cancer, the first step is to find information. Faced with data overload, patients struggle to identify the right knowledge. Accurate cancer diagnosis can reduce the 'paradox of choice'. The way out of this mess is to know your Blue Stage. In a short self-administered prostate cancer staging test, Key walks readers through specific staging information. This book gives patients ideas about options and educates them about step-by-step treatment for prostate cancer.

•Short **STEGEN** exercises will guide you through the appropriate steps and which of the 5 sections of the book to read. • This book consists of seven parts, written by experts in the field of prostate cancer. Five chapters deal with the five stages of cancer.

CHAPTER ONE

Health Problems in Men with Prostate Cancer.

Diagnosis of prostate cancer People often make mistakes. Prostate cancer works in a variety of life-threatening ways. Harmless - related to seeing the same disease at different times. There are actually several types of prostate cancer. Not all diseases are the same. Clinical and pathological stages are important, but not the whole picture. Patients often ask, "Am I stage 1, 2, 3, or 4?" he asks I didn't realize that the old text system was designed to describe the size of a lump (if any) only when the surgeon felt the prostate during a digital rectal exam. Relying on digital research (clinical stage only) is a completely outdated approach! In addition to today's clinical stage, the staging process combines several factors, such as **PSA** level, Gleason score, pathologic stage, scan results, and previous treatment results. Chapter 1 describes how these factors are taken from medical records and combined to determine the risk period. Readers who want a more extensive overview of the five stages of heaven at this time can skip it.

Treatment Measures.

The purpose of this book is to find the best treatment for a man's cancer profile. Adherence to the basics should introduce four broad categories of treatment: observational therapy, topical therapy, systemic therapy, and combination therapy.

Control

Surveillance, also known as "active surveillance," is the process

of controlling cancer without immediate medical intervention. Over the past 20 years, millions of men have been treated for benign prostate cancer. Active surveillance has become increasingly popular with a better understanding of how low-risk (heavenly) prostate cancer behaves. Topical treatment as "prostate targeted therapy strategies" For example, surgical interventions (radical prostatectomy),
radioactive seed injection, external beam type of radiation therapy (IMRT, Proton, CyberKnife) and cryosurgery. Furthermore, a department-only "focus" option was developed. The gland, especially the area where the tumor is located, is treated. Local and focus option
when managed by experienced predecessors perts, large enough to remove the

cancer from the gland degree of consistency.

Systemic Treatment

The greatest risk for prostate cancer is its potential to spread outside the prostate. In the early stages, metastatic disease is microscopic. After a certain period of time, it increases in size and metastases are detected during the scan. Men with microscopic or visible metastases require systemic therapy to circulate the blood and treat the cancer throughout the body. Examples of systemic treatments include hormone therapy, chemotherapy, immunotherapy, and more recently, a new type of radiation therapy that circulates in the blood called Xofigo.

Combined Therapy

The combination of topical and systemic therapies or the simultaneous use of several systemic therapies is called "combination therapy". Improvements in survival have been reported when combination therapy is given to men with advanced or advanced prostate cancer. When considering combination therapy aimed at improving survival, the survival benefit must be weighed against the likelihood of major adverse events. The prostate world is a multi-billion dollar industry that offers powerful financial and professional incentives against the interests of patients.

The process of choosing a treatment can be complex. However, the difficult problem can be broken down into manageable parts. There are too few full-time prostate cancer specialists to handle the 160,000 new cases in the United States each year. Therefore, it is important for patients and their families to educate themselves and manage their treatment plans.

Pathological Stage

A pathology report is a medical document prepared by a pathologist. The report based the diagnosis on the pathologist's examination of a tissue sample taken from the patient's tumor. By viewing and examining the tumor tissue, the pathologist can determine: The cancer is malignant, which means it can grow and spread to other parts of the body. Your doctor will receive these test results when they are available. Ask your doctor to explain the results and the meaning of the pathology report. Description of the microscope this is the most technical part of the report. Describe what cancer cells look like when viewed under a microscope. This section lists several factors that affect diagnosis and treatment. Is the cancer invasive? Most types of tumors can be non-invasive (ie "in place") or invasive. Invasive tumors can spread to other parts of the body through a process called metastasis. Noninvasive tumors do not spread, but may grow or become invasive in the future. For invasive tumors, it is important for the pathologist to record how close the tumor has grown to the healthy tissue. The painting. The classes describe how cancer cells look compared to healthy cells. Typically, pathologists look for differences in the size, shape, and color characteristics of the cells. Tumors with cells that look like healthy cells are called "low-grade" or "well-differentiated" tumors. Tumors with cells that do not resemble healthy cells are called "high-grade," "hypo differentiated," or "undifferentiated." In general, the lower the grade of the tumor, the better the prognosis. Different methods are used to classify different types of cancer. Learn more about the assessment of certain types of cancer. The rate of cell division, the rate of mitosis. Pathologists usually record how many cells are dividing. This is called the mitotic rate. Tumors with few dividing cells are usually low grade, tumor boundaries. Another important factor is whether there are cancer cells at the edge or margin of the biopsy sample. A "positive" or "affected" margin means that the cancer cells are in the margin. This means that cancer cells may still be present in the body lymph nodes. The pathologist also determines whether the cancer has spread to nearby lymph nodes or other organs. Lymph nodes are small pea-shaped organs that help fight disease. If the nodule is cancerous, it is said to be 'positive', otherwise it is said to be 'negative'. Tumors that have spread to the blood or lymph vessels are more likely to spread elsewhere. When the pathologist sees it, they add it to the report.

Questions for the medical team

To better understand the meaning of the pathology report, we recommend asking your medical team the following questions:
What type of cancer do I have and where did it start?
What is the size of the tumor?

Is the cancer invasive or non-invasive?
How fast do cancer cells grow?

What is the grade of the cancer?

What this means?

Is the cancer completely gone?

Are there traces of cancer cells on the edge of the sample?

Are there cancer cells in the lymph or blood vessels?

Clinical/ Observational Stage

A clinical trial is the final step in a long process that begins with research in a laboratory. Before using new treatments in humans in clinical trials, researchers spend years understanding their effects on cancer cells in the laboratory and in animals. They also try to identify any side effects it may cause.

Clinical trials help doctors find new ways to improve the quality of life and treatments for people with certain conditions. Researchers design cancer clinical trials to test new methods. Before using new treatments in humans in clinical trials, researchers spend years understanding how they work on cancer cells in the lab and in animals. Whenever you or a loved one needs cancer treatment, you should consider a clinical trial. Ask your doctor about clinical trials that may be an option for you. At each trial, the person in charge (usually a doctor) is called the chief investigator. The research director creates a research plan called a protocol.

New treatments are being tested in clinical trials.

This summary describes the treatments studied in clinical trials. Not all new treatments under disquisition can be listed. Information about clinical trials is available on the NCI website. Cryosurgery is a treatment that uses tools to indurate and destroy prostate cancer cells. Ultrasound is used to determine the area to be treated. This type of treatment is also called cryotherapy. Cryosurgery can beget erectile dysfunction and leakage of urine from the bladder or coprolite from the rectum. High Intensity concentrated Ultrasound Therapy High- intensity concentrated ultrasound remedy is a treatment that uses ultrasound (high- energy sound swells) to destroy cancer cells. An intrarectal inquiry is used to produce sound swells to treat prostate cancer. Proton radiotherapy Proton radiotherapy is a type of high- energy external radiation remedy that uses a sluice of protons (small appreciatively charged patches) to kill cancer cells. This type of treatment minimizes radiation damage to healthy towel around the excrescence. Photodynamic therapy a cancer treatment that uses medicines and certain types of ray shafts to kill cancer cells. The inactive medicine is fitted into a tone before exposure. The medicine accumulates more in cancer cells than in normal cells. Also, a fiberglass tube is used to deliver the ray light to the cancer cells. In cancer cells, the medicine is actuated and kills the cells. Photodynamic remedy reduces damage to healthy towel. It's substantially used to treat excrescences under the skin or on the mucous membranes of internal organs.

Man Vs Prostrate

CHAPTER TWO

Complete nutrition for knee health and recovery

The modern diet is high in animal protein, fats, and chemicalized food. Excesses of these foods also leads to inflammation, which plays a role in atherosclerosis. Our body is designed to consume a predominantly plant-based, whole foods diet occasionally enhanced with small quantities of animal protein. Contrary to what most people believe, an adult's daily protein requirement is not very high. By consuming a variety of quality vegetable proteins, one can easily meet their daily requirements.

10 foods that are bad for prostate health

If you have prostate disease, avoiding these 10 foods can support prostate health and improve symptoms.

In many cases, not taking it in the first place can prevent prostate disease. Here are 10 foods to avoid that are bad for prostate health.

1. *Alcohol*

Excessive alcohol consumption has many health effects, one of which is prostate health problems.

Research shows that alcohol increases the severity of lower urinary tract symptoms. These include weak urination, incomplete emptying of the bladder and difficulty starting to urinate.

Alcohol's diuretic properties make this type of drink even worse for prostate patients. Therefore, it is recommended not to drink excessively or to stop drinking.

Some research suggests that light alcohol consumption may benefit prostate health. This is because red wine and other alcohols raise HDL levels. It's not alcohol, its high HDL, which improves cardiovascular function and prostate health (1).

2 .*Eggs*

For years we thought that the cholesterol in eggs was bad for our health. New scientific evidence has shown that dietary cholesterol has little effect on serum cholesterol. However, other ingredients in eggs may harm the prostate in the long term. A recent study found that choline in eggs and its metabolite betadine increase the risk of fatal prostate cancer. High choline intake can increase the risk of developing prostate cancer by up to 70%. In fact, choline is not only abundant in eggs. Milk and meat are also abundant sources. So it's not the only food, it's the diet we want to avoid.

In general, a diet rich in fruits and vegetables can prevent this problem. The Mediterranean diet, for example. This diet has positive effects on prostate and heart disease, especially if it includes cruciferous vegetables.

3. *Caffeine*

The problem with caffeine is similar to alcohol. Both have diuretic properties and increase urine production. Caffeine also stimulates the urinary tract, causing additional symptoms not affected by alcohol.

Therefore, patients with urinary tract symptoms should avoid drinks and foods containing caffeine. These drinks include coffee, certain herbal teas, and sports drinks.

It is known to increase urinary incontinence, urination volume, and urination frequency. Preliminary research also suggests that caffeine increases testosterone and levels in the ventral and dorsolateral regions of the prostate.

4. *Spicy Food*

People with urinary problems should avoid foods that are spicy for the prostate.

Caffeine is a mild diuretic and stimulates the urinary tract, but peppers and spicy foods are more irritating. They can worsen all urinary symptoms, especially urgency and incontinence.

Some ingredients in spicy foods, especially capsaicin, may benefit the prostate. However, eating whole foods with the rest of the stimulants is not recommended.

Alternatively, you can reduce bladder intolerance by taking a prostate supplement and avoiding spicy foods.

5. Saturated Fats

In general, eating foods high in saturated fat is not recommended. Prostate health is not an option in this case. Saturated fats are highly inflammatory. Not only does it promote inflammation, it also produces the most aggressive types of inflammatory cytokines. We know that cancer causes inflammation, and this is true. It uses inflammation to grow and nourish new prostate cells. So it's no wonder that saturated fat increases the risk of prostate cancer.

Studies show that a diet high in saturated fat increases the aggressiveness of prostate cancer. In other words, these patients have a dangerous disease in which prostate cancer progresses rapidly.

The prostate grows faster and is more likely to spread. Therefore, avoid foods like bacon and sausages, biscuits, cakes, butter and cream.

6. *Sodium*

People who prefer foods high in sodium to make them taste better have a higher risk of developing prostate-related symptoms. Recent studies have shown that it increases urinary symptoms such as decreased urination and incomplete urination.

Retention symptoms can also worsen, making you urinate more often and causing nocturia. Ideally, you should avoid sodium and use herbs instead. They are safe and offer additional benefits such as sodium-free anti-inflammatory and antioxidant compounds.

7 *Cheese*

This is bad news for dairy lovers because there are at least two components in dairy that can harm your prostate in the long run. This also applies to milk and cheese. Eating cheese at the same time increases calcium and choline intake. Except for these two ingredients, most cheeses are made with whole milk. Therefore, it also contains saturated fat.

Also, we all know that salty cheese has more sodium because it tastes better. In theory, cheese contains many of the above ingredients in a small package and should increase the risk of prostate cancer.

Many studies show this to be true, but it only affects a small number of people. So if you want to make sure your prostate is safe, avoid cheese as one of the 10 worst foods for prostate health

8. *Red Meat*

Raw and processed meats have become a global problem due to the increase in cancer cases. High consumption of red meat is considered a risk factor for prostate cancer.

Many studies talk about carcinogens in red meat. It is activated or formed depending on the cooking method. Cooked, well-cooked and deep-fried red meat has the highest risk of prostate cancer.

The reason is unclear, but it may be due to the heterocyclic amines present in red meat during cooking. Unlike this type of meat, poultry does not have the same effect, and fish has a protective effect because it is rich in omega-3 fatty acids

9. *Processed foods*

It is true that processed foods increase the risk of many types of cancer. One of them is prostate cancer.

The proteus study assessed the incidence of prostate and other cancers and consumption of processed foods, mainly processed red meat, based on data collected in Montreal, Canada between 2005 and 2012. In other words, the more processed foods you eat, the more likely you are to get prostate cancer.

Processed foods include fast food, convenience food, canned goods, microwave dinners, commercial beverages, hams, sausage rolls, cookies and cakes, pastries, and cereals.

10. *Salad Dressing*

Salad dressings in utmost cases aren't useful. Utmost fall under the order of reused foods because they're packaged and filled with chemicals. They're also frequently high in swab and impregnated fat. Thus, there's nothing useful in marketable salads. Sauces and olive oil painting can be used rather. They give anti-inflammatory and antioxidant composites that are salutary for prostate and overall health. Conclusion Prostate towel naturally expands as we progress. Still, not all of us have symptoms of BPH. So having a healthy prostate is not about heredity or age. It also depends on what you eat. This composition describes the 10 worst foods to avoid to reduce your threat of prostate cancer and BPH. In addition to medical advice, avoiding these foods can reduce the rush of prostate cancer. The list begins with diuretic foods and bladder instigations that worsen urinary symptoms similar as alcohol, caffeine, and racy foods. Now you know that choline in eggs, impregnated adipose acids and sodium in salty foods are bad for the prostate. Dairy products, especially rubbish, increase the threat of prostate problems, so red meat consumption should be reduced. Packaged and reused foods, including salad dressings, should be avoided under all circumstances. Diet and life play an important part in precluding prostate problems and managing symptoms if they formerly exist. So eat right, exercise and follow your croaker's advice. However, you may not need prostate cancer treatment or the annoying symptoms of BPH in the future, if you take care of yourself moment.

Man Vs Prostrate

CHAPTER THREE

The Relationship between Physical Activity and BPH

By now, we've heard about the value of exercise in staying healthy. Hundreds of studies spanning more than half a century show that regular exercise reduces the risk of several fatal problems, including heart disease, stroke, and some cancers (such as colon cancer). It also reduces the effects of chronic conditions such as high blood pressure, diabetes and arthritis. Surprisingly, regular exercise can actually help prevent some prostate diseases and improve prostate health. New scientific evidence suggests that a few hours of exercise a week can help control an enlarged prostate.

Evaluation of the evidence

Relatively few studies have investigated the relationship between physical activity and

BPH, a condition that causes an enlarged prostate, frequent urination, poor urine flow, and other symptoms. One of the first articles published in 1998 was based on data from a survey of 30,634 men participating in a follow-up study by health professionals, of whom 3,743 had BPH. Researchers have found an inverse relationship between physical activity and BPH symptoms. Simply put, physically active men are less likely to develop BPH. Low- to moderate-intensity physical activity, such as regular walking at a moderate pace, has also been shown to be beneficial. The researchers found that walking three more hours per week was associated with an additional 10% lower risk.

The researchers also found that men who watched the most TV and video (>41 hours per week) were twice as likely to develop BPH symptoms as those who watched the least (5 hours or less). Interestingly, the more time you spent watching TV on the couch, the more cases of BPH occurred, regardless of exercise time.

Other studies have reached less conclusive conclusions. For example, a physician's health study based on 320 cases found that men who were relatively sedentary had a lower risk of BPH than men who were more active. However, completely sedentary men had a higher risk of BPH.

To further investigate the relationship between physical activity and BPH, Italian researchers analyzed the occupational and recreational activity levels of 1,369 men with BPH and 1,451 without BPH. Men in physically active occupations, such as farmers and construction workers, are 30 to 40 percent less likely to develop BPH than white-collar men. Exercise helped too. Men who exercise more than 5 hours per week are 30 to 50% less likely to develop BPH than men who exercise less than 2 hours per week. Men with the highest levels of occupational and recreational physical activity are 60% less likely to develop the condition. (To read all of these studies in person, see "HBP Exercises and Studies" below.)

What is the connection? No one knows for sure, but researchers say that high levels of physical activity may decrease testosterone, which regulates prostate growth and promote the development of BPH. Another explanation is that exercise reduces the activity of the sympathetic nervous system, the part of the nervous system that is activated during stress, thereby reducing the severity of urinary tract symptoms.

Take Advantage of It
How Much Exercise Should I Do If I'm Concerned about My Prostate Health?

What activities can you do? Should i run how many hours should I spend on the treadmill at the gym to rest and breathe for a healthy prostate? There is no specific exercise program for men who are concerned about BPH. However, a comprehensive exercise program of 30 minutes of exercise throughout the week or most days of the week can have a profound effect on your health. And you don't have to do it right away. It can be divided into three 10-minute parts. Aim for moderate speed. Top tip: When you practice, you should be able to carry on a conversation. Yes, short sentences are good too. If your breathing is too heavy for a comfortable conversation, take a step back. As the activity becomes easier, increase the duration or pace of the exercise.

If you wish, you can run or use the treadmill in the gym (see "Health Club" below). But don't forget to ride your bike (see "Saddle and Bike Health" below), swim, or jog. In fact, walking has been hailed as the perfect form of exercise because it can be done by people of all ages and fitness levels. Walking is also safe for almost everyone. It won't damage your joints or raise your heart rate to dangerous levels, even in people with poor health.

What Is My Heart Rate?

Many people have learned to measure their heart rate during aerobic exercise to make sure they are reaching their target heart rate. To calculate your maximum heart rate, subtract your age from 220. Multiply the result by 50% for the lower end of the target range or 75% for the upper end. However, this technique has its drawbacks. Few people have an accurate heart rate. When you're not exercising, your heart rate drops so quickly that measuring it after you stop won't tell you your true level of exercise. Paying attention to your body's cues, such as how hard you're breathing, can tell you if you can work harder or slower.

Smart Fitness Club

You don't have to be a member of a health club to exercise. Registering as a member offers several benefits. A variety of equipment and training sessions are available, making it easy to change up your routine and avoid boredom. Your personal trainer will create a routine and teach you how to use the equipment correctly. Many people find that going to the gym motivates them to work out more often to earn their money. On the other hand, some insurance companies cover some or all of the costs, but membership is often expensive. Also, some gyms can be so crowded that you can't attend the classes you want or wait in line to use your equipment. You have to visit the gym often to find out what the atmosphere is like. Make sure the location and time fits your schedule. If you would like to work with a trainer on a regular basis, please ask about additional fees and trainer qualifications. Find trainers certified by a professional body like the American College of Sports Medicine.

Bicycle Saddle and Health

When you ride for a long time on a narrow bicycle seat, the nerves in the perineum, the area between the testicles and the anus, are compressed, causing tingling in the penis. Erectile dysfunction is rare. Problems can persist for a week to a month after a long bike ride. You can avoid these problems by taking the following precautions:

Choose a spacious area with plenty of padding.
Find a gel-filled, anatomically friendly spot.

Wear padded cycling shorts. Do not tilt the seat forward. This increases the pressure on the perineum. Make sure the seat height is correct. Do not fully extend your legs at the bottom of the pedal stroke. Raise the handle and stand up straight.

Make sure the top of the frame is at least 2 inches below your shoulders. If you fall, cover the band with a pad to protect your genitals.

Whatever activity you choose (see "Choose Your Favorites" below for ideas), avoid random, high-intensity combat. First, the health benefits of exercise are based on total amount, not intensity. Most importantly, vigorous exercise increases the chances of sudden death from muscle or joint damage and cardiac arrhythmias. This is especially true if you are a "weekend warrior" or have not had a medical checkup to prevent serious illness.

Aerobic Exercise - Pick Your Favorite Activities

The following tasks: walking Boost" dozens of activities with aerobic exercise. Choose one or more that you like. Enjoying your daily routine increases your chances of continuing your training. Consider

Hiking

Raking leaves

Gardening

Aerobics

Bicycling

Dancing

Swimming

Jogging/running

Golfing

Tennis

Racquetball

Rowing

Before starting aerobic exercise, warm up for 5-10 minutes with light stretches and low-intensity exercises. This is very important to avoid injury. Also use a cool down of the same length.

In addition to aerobic exercise such as walking, a comprehensive exercise program that includes strength exercises, flexibility exercises (stretching exercises), and balance exercises; each benefits the body in different ways. Strength training builds muscle and bone and improves the body's muscle mass ratio. Flexibility exercises help stretch muscles, keep joints supple and prevent injuries. Balance exercises can help prevent falls, which can lead to injury.

Exercise safely

Lack of exercise is more harmful to people than excessive exercise." While the benefits of regular exercise far outweigh the risks, there are risks that range from minor discomfort to life-threatening conditions. The most common risk associated with exercise is likely to be muscle and joint problems. It can be caused by quick movements such as catching a tennis ball, sprains, tears or breaks. Stiffness, joint and muscle pain, and inflammation of tendons and ligaments can occur when you exercise too hard or too often, use improper techniques or equipment (such as worn-out sneakers), increase your activity level too quickly, or don't bounce back. Low levels of exercise after periods of normal inactivity.

The greatest risk associated with exercise is sudden

Death. Sedentary people who suddenly start vigorous exercise can increase their chances of dying from a heart attack or arrhythmia, a change in the heartbeat. But it's important to keep this in perspective. The absolute risk of sudden death among all exercise episodes is very small - 1 in 1.51 million exercises. It is important to note that the risk of sudden death discussed here is associated with vigorous exercise. If you exercise at a moderate level, the risk is low.

To make exercise as safe and enjoyable as possible, follow these simple precautions: Talk to your doctor before starting an exercise program, especially if you have health problems. He can help you determine your limits and create a routine that fits your fitness level.
Preheat and cool properly. Drink plenty of fluids.

Watch out for signs of heat stroke (headaches, dizziness, nausea, fainting, convulsions or palpitations), especial ly in hot and humid weather. If possible, plan to exercise early in the morning or in the evening when temperatures drop. Do not exercise when you are sick. When you recover, keep exercising, but give yourself time to get back to normal. Record your injuries. However, this does not mean that you should stop exercising. For example, if you sprained your ankle while running, try swimming or other exercises that use your arms and hold your toes. Wear loose, comfortable clothing that is appropriate for the weather. Be aware of your surroundings. For example, if you are walking or running, you should always be aware of traffic jams. If you are cycling, follow the traffic jams. Don't forget to wear a helmet and follow the traffic rules. You are walking down a brightly lit street. Consider bringing your cell phone. The most important thing is to listen to your body. Don't overload yourself. Discontinue if you are unable to complete an exercise session, cannot carry on a conversation during exercise, feel weak after exercise, or have joint pain. If you experience burning, tingling or fullness in your chest or upper body, stop the activity and seek medical attention immediately. Fainting or loss of consciousness; wheezing or difficulty breathing that lasts more than a few minutes; or bone or joint pain.

CHAPTER FOUR

Prostate Health Supplements - What Are the Common Ingredients?

Supplements do not cure or cure prostate problems. However, many people claim that it helps prevent or reduce symptoms associated with prostate problems by reducing inflammation in general. Ingredients commonly used in supplements

Overall, the evidence supporting the effectiveness of supplements for prostate health is weak.

However, limited research suggests that certain ingredients may help reduce uncomfortable symptoms associated with prostate problems. Some ingredients may help make you more comfortable, while others may be ineffective or potentially harmful to prostate health. Therefore, it is important to always consult your doctor before taking any prostate supplement

Saw Palmetto (Serenoa repens) is one of the most common ingredients in prostate supplements. It is a palm tree native to the southeastern United States (8). Specifically, saw palmetto fruit and extracts help treat urinary tract symptoms associated with BPH. The exact mechanism is not known, but saw palmetto's anti-inflammatory effect is thought to play a role. In a study of 165 men with BPH, taking 160 mg of saw palmetto extract capsules 4 times daily for 12 weeks significantly improved prostate symptoms, urinary flow, and quality of life.

Although promising, research on the effects of saw palmetto on BPH symptoms in humans is limited. There are also mixed studies on its effectiveness on BPH symptoms.

In addition, the optimal effective dose for patients with BPH is unclear, as doses vary widely between studies (9). Also, because most studies only included people diagnosed with BPH or other prostate problems, it's unclear whether supplements can help prevent prostate-related urinary tract symptoms in healthy adults.

Saw palmetto extract may also help prevent prostate cancer. Some evidence from test-tube and animal studies suggests that saw palmetto treatment may help inhibit the proliferation and growth of prostate cancer cells.

However, this protective effect has not been demonstrated in humans. Overall, more research is needed to confirm the potential benefits and appropriate doses of saw palmetto extract for prostate health.

Finally, although it is generally considered safe, some people may not tolerate bipalmetto well. The most commonly reported side effects are headache, dizziness, nausea, constipation, and allergic reactions.

Beta-Sitosterol

Beta-sitosterols are common plant compounds that belong to many groups of compounds called plant sterols. Plant sterols produced from plants are natural steroids with health benefits, including lowering cholesterol.

In particular, beta-sitosterol has been shown to have powerful antioxidant and anti-inflammatory properties (18, 19). Additionally, the beta-sitosterol found in saw palmetto has been studied for its ability to reduce inflammation associated with BPH urinary symptoms and prevent prostate cancer.

Although limited test-tube and animal studies suggest that beta-sitosterol has potential anticancer effects, more human studies are needed. A review examining dietary intake of plant sterols, including beta-sitosterol, and cancer risk found that total plant sterol intake was associated with reduced cancer risk (21).

However, it is not known whether plant sterol supplements have the same protective effect. Regarding their role in BPH, a study in 91 men with symptoms of BPH compared the effects of beta-sitosterol-rich saw palmetto oil and saw palmetto oil alone.

Studies have shown that the fortified oil was significantly more effective than saw palmetto oil or a placebo in reducing the severity of urinary tract symptoms over 12 weeks. Again, despite the promising results, much more research is needed on the effectiveness and optimal dosage of beta-sitosterol for prostate health.

Pollen Extract

Chronic prostatitis is a serious disease involving inflammation of the prostate. This condition is more common in men under the age of 50 and is often characterized by pelvic pain, sexual dysfunction, and difficulty urinating and ejaculating.

Although anti-inflammatory drugs like aspirin and ibuprofen are commonly used to reduce inflammation and pain, there is growing interest in using pollen extracts as natural alternatives to these drugs. In a study of 65 patients with chronic prostatitis, taking capsules containing 1 gram of pollen extract and various **B** vitamins daily for 3 months significantly improved symptoms of chronic prostatitis

In addition, the pollen extract group was found to have significantly lower levels of interleukin 8 (IL-8), a higher inflammatory marker, in patients with chronic prostatitis. Similarly, a review of 10 studies found that pollen extract significantly improved quality of life and symptom scores in people diagnosed with chronic prostatitis.

The most commonly used pollen extract mixture used in this clinical trial is Graminex, a standardized extract mixture of rye pollen (Secal grain), corn pollen (Zea mays), and timothy pollen (Phleum pratense) . Reviews also found pollen extracts to be safe with no dangerous side effects.

Pygeum

Herbal extract derived from the bark of the African cherry tree (Prunus africana), is another common ingredient found in prostate supplements. Limited test-tube and human studies suggest that pygeum extract may reduce inflammation associated with prostatitis and prevent the growth of cancer cells.

A previous review of 18 studies investigated the benefits of pygeum supplementation in improving BPH-related symptoms compared to placebo. According to reviews, pygeum supplementation significantly improved urinary flow. Additionally, men who used pygeum were twice as likely to report an improvement in overall symptoms.

Nettle Root

Stinging nettle (Urtica dioica) is a flowering plant widely used in alternative medicine to reduce pain and inflammation.

It has been shown to contain several plant compounds with powerful antioxidant, anti-inflammatory and antibacterial effects. It is commonly found in supplements used for urinary tract and bladder infections.

Limited animal and human studies suggest that it may help reduce lower urinary tract symptoms associated with BPH. A six-month study in 558 adult men with symptomatic BPH found that taking

120 mg of stinging nettle root extract three times daily significantly improved lower urinary tract symptoms compared to placebo.

Additionally, test-tube and animal studies have shown that nettle root may have anti-cancer properties. However, there are currently no studies supporting its ability to prevent prostate cancer in humans.

Despite promising results, most studies on nettle root extract for prostate health are limited and outdated. Larger studies are needed to evaluate the role of BPH in prostate cancer, as well as whether it can reduce symptoms associated with BPH.

Pumpkin Seed Oil

Due to its high concentration of anti-inflammatory compounds, pumpkin seed oil is another common ingredient in prostate supplement. By reducing inflammation, pumpkin seed oil is thought to help improve urinary tract symptoms associated with BPH and chronic nonbacterial prostatitis

In a study of 60 men with BPH, taking 350 mg of natural pumpkin seed oil extract and 500 mg of fat-free hydroethanolic pumpkin seed extract equivalent to 10 grams of pumpkin seeds significantly reduced symptoms for 12 weeks. In particular, consumption of pumpkin seed extract has been shown to reduce the International Prostate Symptom Score by an average of 30.

However, research on the effectiveness and optimal dosage of pumpkin seed oil for prostate problems is generally limited.

Vitamin D

Vitamin D is an essential nutrient required for many important processes in the body, including immune function and bone health

Several observational studies have also suggested an association between low vitamin D levels and an increased risk of prostate cancer. However, research on whether vitamin D supplementation can prevent prostate cancer is inconclusive. One review found an increased risk of prostate cancer in people with high levels of vitamin D Taking vitamin D supplements may be beneficial for men who are vitamin D deficient or deficient, but high-dose supplements are not currently recommended for prostate health.

Zinc

Zinc is an essential mineral that plays an important role in cell growth and DNA repair.

Interestingly, studies have shown that men with prostate cancer have significantly decreased levels of zinc in their prostate. Therefore, research is ongoing into the potential role of zinc in preventing or slowing the growth of prostate cancer

While some studies have shown that high zinc intake is associated with a reduced risk of developing prostate cancer, other studies have shown that zinc intake is associated with an increased risk of prostate cancer. In general, studies on zinc and prostate cancer are inconclusive. Therefore, zinc supplements are not recommended for prostate health unless prescribed by a healthcare professional. Vitamin E

Vitamin E is another important nutrient often found in prostate supplements.

Some older studies have shown that vitamin E's antioxidant properties may prevent prostate cancer. However, recent studies have linked vitamin E supplementation with an increased risk of prostate cancer.

The Selenium and Vitamin E Cancer Prevention Trial (SELECT) was a large trial in which 35,533 men were randomized to one of four treatments. 200 mcg daily selenium, 400 IU vitamin E, 400 IU vitamin E + 200 mcg. Intake of selenium or placebo per day. At the end of the study, men who only took vitamin E supplements had a significantly higher risk of developing prostate cancer over a 7-year period.

While research into a possible link between vitamin E and prostate cancer continues, vitamin E supplements are not currently recommended to reduce the risk of prostate cancer. Men should avoid vitamin E supplements unless recommended by their healthcare provider.

Selenium

Selenium is another important mineral that has sparked controversy over its safety and effectiveness for prostate health. In two large reviews, high levels of selenium in the body were associated with a reduced risk of prostate cancer, especially in current and former smokers.

However, one study of 4,459 men found that selenium intake after a prostate cancer diagnosis was associated with an increased risk of death from prostate cancer.(Another study raised concerns about selenium supplementation because it found that consuming 200 mcg of selenium supplementation daily increased the risk of prostate cancer in men with high baseline levels of selenium before supplementation.

However, selenium supplementation has not been shown to have a significant effect (positive or negative) on prostate cancer risk in people with low baseline selenium levels. Overall, more research is needed on the safety and effectiveness of selenium supplementation, especially in populations with high selenium levels and diagnosed with prostate cancer.

To fall into

Many prostate supplements on the market support prostate health.

Some ingredients may improve urinary symptoms associated with prostate problems, but research on their effectiveness is generally limited. It's also important to pay close attention to what the products you buy contain, as some supplements may contain ingredients such as vitamin E or zinc, which can be harmful to prostate health.

When buying supplements, you should always choose products from reputable companies. To ensure quality and accuracy, look for third-party certified products from organizations such as **NSF** International or the United States Pharmacopeia (**USP**).

Finally, it is important to discuss prostate health issues with your doctor, as supplements cannot or will not cure prostate problems. In particular, any symptoms of prostate cancer should be discussed with your doctor as soon as possible.

Man Vs Prostrate

CHAPTER 5

Frequently Asked Question about Prostrate Cancer

What is the life expectancy of a man with prostate cancer?

Life expectancy: Almost 100% of men with early prostate cancer live more than 5 years after diagnosis. Men with advanced prostate cancer or cancer that has spread to other sites have a lower survival rate. About one-third survive 5 years after diagnosis

How fast does prostate cancer spread?

Prostate cancer is a slow-growing cancer that is often confined to the prostate and requires little or no treatment. In some cases, it can take up to 8 years for the prostate to spread to other parts of the body (metastasize), usually the bones.

Risk Factors for Prostate Cancer

Age

Prostate cancer is rare in men under the age of 40, but the risk of prostate cancer increases dramatically after age 50. Six out of 10 cases of prostate cancer occur in men over the age of 65.

Race/Ethnicity

Prostate cancer is more common in African-American men and Afro-Caribbean men than in other races. And when it occurs in men, it is usually younger. Prostate cancer is less common among Asian Americans and Hispanic/Hispanic men than among non-Hispanic whites. The reasons for these racial and ethnic differences are unclear.

Geography

Prostate cancer is more common in North America, northwestern Europe, Australia, and the Caribbean. It is rare in Asia, Africa, Central and South America.

The reason is not clear. More intensive prostate cancer screening in some developed countries explains at least some of these differences, but other factors, such as differences in lifestyle (such as diet), may also be important. For example, Asian Americans have a lower risk of prostate cancer than white Americans, but the risk is higher than Asian men. Family History Prostate cancer runs in some families and in some cases it can be hereditary or genetic. However, most cases of prostate cancer occur in men with no family history. If a man has a father or brother who has prostate cancer, his risk of getting the disease is doubled. (Men who have a brother who has the disease are at higher risk than men who have a father.) Men with multiple relatives have a much higher risk, especially if they have younger relatives when they are diagnosed with cancer.